COMPLETE GUIDE TO NEPHRECTOMY

Essential Handbook To Kidney Removal, Techniques, Types, Indications, Risks, Recovery, and Post-operative Care

DR. BRUNO HORAN

Copyright © 2023 by Dr. Bruno Horan

Disclaimer:

The information provided in this book, is intended for general informational purposes only and should not be considered as professional advice.

The author has made every effort to ensure the accuracy of the information presented. However, readers are advised to consult with a qualified healthcare professional before attempting any herbal remedies or making significant changes to their wellness routine. Individual health conditions vary, and what may be suitable for one person may not be appropriate for another.

It is important to note that the author is not in any endorsement deal, partnership, or affiliation with any organization, brand, or company mentioned in this book. Any references to specific products or services are based on the author's personal experience or general knowledge and do not imply an endorsement or promotion of those products or services

Contents

ABOUT THIS BOOK

Discover the essential guide to nephrectomy—a comprehensive resource designed to empower individuals facing kidney surgery with knowledge and understanding. Delving into the intricacies of kidney function and anatomy, this book illuminates the vital role kidneys play in our overall health. From exploring common kidney disorders to identifying symptoms that necessitate nephrectomy, each section prepares readers to make informed decisions about their healthcare journey.

Detailed insights into diagnostic tests and different nephrectomy procedures—such as partial, radical, laparoscopic, open, and robotic-assisted—are provided to guide patients in selecting the most suitable approach. Preparation for surgery is meticulously covered, encompassing preoperative evaluations, dietary adjustments, and mental readiness, ensuring patients are well-prepared physically and emotionally.

On surgery day, readers gain a clear understanding of what to expect—from anesthesia options to the step-by-step procedure itself. Post-operative care is meticulously detailed, addressing pain management, monitoring protocols, and rehabilitation strategies, fostering a smooth recovery process.

Potential complications are candidly discussed, along with guidance on recognizing early signs and managing long-term risks. The book also sheds light on life after nephrectomy, offering practical advice on adjusting to a single kidney, long-term health monitoring, and psychological considerations. Common concerns and frequently asked questions are addressed with clarity, providing reassurance and valuable insights.

Looking ahead, the book explores advances in nephrectomy techniques, ongoing research in kidney surgery, and future treatment possibilities, emphasizing continuous improvements in patient outcomes and advocating for increased awareness within the healthcare community.

This comprehensive guide serves not only as a trusted companion through the nephrectomy process but also as a beacon of knowledge, empowering readers to navigate their healthcare decisions with confidence and clarity.

CHAPTER ONE

UNDERSTANDING KIDNEY FUNCTION

The kidneys are essential organs responsible for a range of critical functions that keep the body in balance. These bean-shaped organs, located on either side of the spine just below the rib cage, filter waste products, excess fluids, and toxins from the blood, which are then excreted as urine. Each day, the kidneys filter around 150 quarts of blood, producing about 1 to 2 quarts of urine.

Kidneys also play a pivotal role in maintaining the body's electrolyte balance, regulating sodium, potassium, and calcium levels to ensure proper muscle and nerve function. Additionally, they help manage blood pressure by releasing the enzyme renin, which adjusts blood vessel constriction. The kidneys also produce erythropoietin, a hormone that stimulates red blood cell production in the bone marrow, ensuring adequate oxygen transport throughout the body.

Another critical function of the kidneys is maintaining acid-base balance. They filter and reabsorb bicarbonate from urine and excrete hydrogen ions, preventing acidosis and alkalosis. Furthermore, kidneys activate vitamin D to its usable form, calcitriol, which aids in calcium absorption for bone health. This intricate balance of filtration, secretion, and hormonal activity underscores the kidneys' vital role in overall health.

Anatomy And Function Of The Kidneys

Each kidney is about the size of a large fist, roughly 11-14 cm long, 6 cm wide, and 4 cm thick. They are protected by a layer of adipose tissue and a tough, fibrous capsule. The outer region, called the cortex, contains nephrons—the functional units of the kidney. Each nephron consists of a glomerulus, where blood filtration begins, and a tubule, where reabsorption and secretion occur.

The inner region, the medulla, contains the renal pyramids, where urine collects before draining into the renal pelvis and subsequently the ureter. Blood enters the kidneys through the renal arteries, which branch into smaller arterioles and capillaries within the nephrons. Here, waste products and excess substances are filtered out, while essential nutrients and water are reabsorbed.

The kidneys' structural complexity supports their multifaceted roles. For instance, the glomerulus filters blood at high pressure, allowing small molecules like water, glucose, and electrolytes to pass through while retaining larger molecules such as proteins and blood cells. The tubules then selectively reabsorb useful substances and secrete additional wastes into the urine. This intricate process is fine-tuned by hormones like aldosterone and antidiuretic hormone (ADH), which adjust reabsorption rates based on the body's needs.

Role Of Kidneys In The Body

The kidneys are central to homeostasis, ensuring a stable internal environment despite external changes. They regulate fluid balance by adjusting urine volume and concentration, responding to hydration levels, and conserving water during dehydration or expelling excess fluid when overhydrated.

Blood pressure regulation is another key function. Through the renin-angiotensin-aldosterone system (RAAS), the kidneys respond to low blood pressure by releasing renin, which triggers a cascade that increases blood volume and vessel constriction, raising blood pressure. Conversely, they release atrial natriuretic peptide (ANP) in response to high blood pressure, promoting sodium and water excretion to reduce blood volume.

Kidneys also manage waste elimination, filtering metabolic byproducts like urea, creatinine, and ammonia from the blood. These wastes are the result of protein metabolism and muscle activity, and their accumulation can be toxic if not properly excreted. Additionally, the kidneys help detoxify the body by excreting drugs and environmental toxins.

Another crucial role is in maintaining electrolyte balance. Kidneys adjust the excretion and reabsorption of sodium, potassium, calcium, and magnesium, essential for muscle function, nerve conduction, and bone health. They also regulate acid-base balance, excreting hydrogen ions and reabsorbing bicarbonate to keep blood pH within a narrow range.

Common Kidney Disorders

Several disorders can impair kidney function, leading to serious health issues. Chronic kidney disease (CKD) is a progressive loss of kidney function over time, often caused by diabetes, hypertension, or glomerulonephritis. CKD can lead to end-stage renal disease (ESRD), requiring dialysis or kidney transplantation.

Acute kidney injury (AKI) is a sudden decrease in kidney function, often due to severe dehydration, blood loss, infection, or medications. AKI can be reversible if treated promptly but can lead to chronic issues if not addressed.

Polycystic kidney disease (PKD) is a genetic disorder characterized by the growth of numerous cysts in the kidneys, leading to enlargement and impaired function. PKD can cause pain, hypertension, and kidney failure over time.

Glomerulonephritis is inflammation of the glomeruli, often due to infections, autoimmune diseases, or conditions like lupus. This disorder can lead to hematuria, proteinuria, and reduced kidney function.

Kidney stones are hard deposits of minerals and salts that form in the kidneys. They can cause severe pain, urinary tract infections, and obstructive uropathy if they block urine flow.

Signs And Symptoms Requiring Nephrectomy

Nephrectomy, or the surgical removal of a kidney, is indicated for several conditions. Renal cell carcinoma, the most common type of kidney cancer, often necessitates nephrectomy to prevent the spread of malignancy. Symptoms of kidney cancer include blood in the urine, persistent back or side pain, unexplained weight loss, and fatigue.

Severe kidney damage from trauma, such as a car accident or a fall, may also require nephrectomy if the kidney cannot be repaired. Symptoms of significant kidney injury include abdominal pain, blood in the urine, and decreased urine output.

Recurrent severe kidney infections (pyelonephritis) that do not respond to treatment can lead to chronic kidney damage, necessitating nephrectomy.

Symptoms include fever, chills, flank pain, and recurrent urinary tract infections.

Nephrectomy may be required for large, symptomatic kidney stones that cause persistent pain, hematuria, and urinary obstruction. If the stones cannot be removed through less invasive methods, surgery may be the only option.

Polycystic kidney disease with severe pain, bleeding, or infection, and poor kidney function may also necessitate nephrectomy. Symptoms include chronic back or side pain, blood in the urine, and frequent urinary infections.

Diagnostic Tests Before Nephrectomy

Before a nephrectomy, a series of diagnostic tests are conducted to assess kidney function and overall health. Blood tests, including serum creatinine and blood urea nitrogen (BUN), measure waste products in the blood and evaluate kidney function. Electrolyte levels are also checked to ensure they are within normal ranges.

Imaging tests are critical for visualizing the kidneys and surrounding structures. Ultrasound uses sound waves to create images of the kidneys, identifying tumors, cysts, and stones. CT scans provide detailed cross-sectional images, highlighting the size, shape, and location of kidney abnormalities. MRI offers high-resolution images, particularly useful for soft tissues and identifying tumors.

A renal scan, involving the injection of a radioactive tracer, assesses kidney function and blood flow. It helps determine the function of each kidney separately, crucial for planning a nephrectomy. Angiography, an imaging test that uses contrast dye and X-rays, evaluates blood supply to the kidneys, identifying any vascular issues.

A biopsy, where a small tissue sample is taken from the kidney, may be performed if there is suspicion of cancer or other serious conditions. This helps in diagnosing the type and stage of kidney disease and guiding treatment decisions.

Urinalysis, examining the urine for protein, blood, and other abnormalities, provides additional information on kidney health. This test can indicate infections, inflammation, or the presence of kidney stones.

Preoperative evaluations, including cardiac and respiratory assessments, ensure that the patient is fit for surgery. These evaluations minimize the risk of complications during and after the nephrectomy.

CHAPTER TWO

TYPES OF NEPHRECTOMY PROCEDURES

Nephrectomy, the surgical removal of a kidney, can be performed through various procedures, each tailored to specific medical conditions and patient needs.

The primary types of nephrectomy include partial nephrectomy, radical nephrectomy, laparoscopic nephrectomy, and robotic-assisted nephrectomy. Understanding these types helps patients and medical professionals make informed decisions about the best surgical approach.

Partial Nephrectomy

Partial nephrectomy involves removing only the diseased or damaged portion of the kidney, preserving as much healthy kidney tissue as possible.

This procedure is often preferred for small, localized kidney tumors or other conditions affecting a limited area of the kidney.

The goal is to maintain maximum kidney function while effectively treating the underlying issue. Surgeons employ advanced techniques to ensure precise removal of the affected tissue while minimizing damage to surrounding healthy tissue.

Radical Nephrectomy

Radical nephrectomy entails the complete removal of the kidney, often including surrounding tissues, such as the adrenal gland, lymph nodes, and fatty tissue.

This procedure is typically recommended for larger or more aggressive kidney tumors that cannot be treated effectively with partial nephrectomy.

Radical nephrectomy may also be necessary when the cancer has spread beyond the kidney.

The comprehensive nature of this procedure aims to eliminate the disease and prevent recurrence, although it results in the loss of an entire kidney.

Laparoscopic Vs. Open Nephrectomy

Laparoscopic Nephrectomy

Laparoscopic nephrectomy is a minimally invasive surgical approach where small incisions are made to insert a camera and surgical instruments. The surgeon performs the procedure by viewing the internal organs on a monitor, allowing for precise and less invasive surgery. Benefits of laparoscopic nephrectomy include reduced postoperative pain, shorter hospital stays, quicker recovery, and smaller scars. This method is suitable for both partial and radical nephrectomy, depending on the specific case.

Open Nephrectomy

Open nephrectomy, the traditional approach, involves a larger incision to access the kidney directly. This method provides the surgeon with a clear view and more room to maneuver during complex procedures. Open nephrectomy is often reserved for cases where the tumor is very large, located in a challenging position, or when previous surgeries have caused significant scar tissue. Although it involves a longer recovery period and more postoperative discomfort compared to laparoscopic nephrectomy, it remains a vital option for specific clinical scenarios.

Robotic-Assisted Nephrectomy

Robotic-assisted nephrectomy is an advanced form of minimally invasive surgery utilizing a robotic system to enhance the surgeon's precision, dexterity, and control. The robotic system consists of multiple arms equipped with surgical instruments and a high-definition 3D camera. The surgeon operates from a console, controlling the robotic arms with exact movements. This technique allows for highly precise dissection and suturing, reducing the risk of complications and improving outcomes. Robotic-assisted nephrectomy can be used for both partial and radical nephrectomy, offering the benefits of minimally invasive surgery with enhanced precision.

Choosing The Right Procedure

Selecting the appropriate nephrectomy procedure depends on various factors, including the size, location, and nature of the kidney condition, the patient's overall health, and the surgeon's expertise. A thorough evaluation by a multidisciplinary medical team, including urologists, oncologists, and radiologists, is essential to determine the most suitable approach.

Considerations include the potential for preserving kidney function, the likelihood of complete tumor removal, recovery time, and potential risks and benefits of each procedure.

Patients should engage in detailed discussions with their healthcare providers, asking questions and understanding the rationale behind the recommended surgical approach.

By weighing the options and understanding the specifics of each type of nephrectomy, patients can make informed decisions that align with their health goals and treatment preferences.

CHAPTER THREE

PREPARING FOR NEPHRECTOMY

Preoperative Evaluation And Tests

Before undergoing a nephrectomy, a thorough preoperative evaluation is essential to ensure the surgery is as safe and effective as possible.

This evaluation typically includes a variety of tests and assessments to gauge your overall health and the functionality of your kidneys.

Medical History Review: Your healthcare team will begin by reviewing your complete medical history, including any previous surgeries, existing medical conditions, and current medications. This information helps identify any potential risks or complications that may arise during surgery.

Physical Examination: A comprehensive physical examination will be conducted to assess your general health and identify any physical conditions that may affect the surgery. This examination often includes measuring your blood pressure, heart rate, and respiratory function.

Blood Tests: Blood tests are crucial in evaluating your kidney function and overall health. Common tests include a complete blood count (CBC), electrolyte levels, and renal function tests such as serum creatinine and blood urea nitrogen (BUN) levels.

Imaging Studies: Imaging studies, such as an ultrasound, CT scan, or MRI, are used to visualize the kidneys and surrounding structures. These images help the surgical team plan the procedure by providing detailed information about the size, shape, and location of the kidneys and any potential abnormalities.

Electrocardiogram (ECG): An ECG is performed to assess your heart's electrical activity and identify any potential cardiac issues that need to be addressed before surgery.

Pulmonary Function Tests: If you have a history of respiratory problems, pulmonary function tests may be conducted to evaluate your lung function and ensure you can tolerate the anesthesia and surgical procedure.

Dietary And Lifestyle Preparations

Preparing your body for nephrectomy involves making specific dietary and lifestyle adjustments to optimize your health and minimize surgical risks.

Healthy Diet: In the weeks leading up to your surgery, focus on eating a balanced diet rich in fruits, vegetables, lean proteins, and whole grains.

Avoid processed foods, excessive sugars, and high-fat foods to maintain optimal health and support your immune system.

Hydration: Staying well-hydrated is crucial for maintaining kidney function and overall health. Drink plenty of water each day, unless otherwise directed by your healthcare team, to ensure your body is well-prepared for surgery.

Alcohol and Tobacco: Avoid alcohol and tobacco use in the weeks before your surgery. Alcohol can interfere with anesthesia and medications, while smoking can impair lung function and slow the healing process.

Exercise: Regular physical activity can help improve your cardiovascular health and overall fitness, making it easier for your body to recover from surgery. Aim for at least 30 minutes of moderate exercise most days of the week, unless advised otherwise by your doctor.

Weight Management: If you are overweight, your healthcare team may recommend losing weight before surgery. Even a small amount of weight loss can reduce surgical risks and improve recovery outcomes.

Medications And Supplements Guidelines

Managing your medications and supplements correctly is critical in the days and weeks leading up to nephrectomy to avoid complications and ensure a smooth surgical process.

Current Medications: Provide your healthcare team with a complete list of all medications you are currently taking, including prescription drugs, over-the-counter medications, and herbal supplements. Some medications may need to be adjusted or temporarily discontinued before surgery.

Blood Thinners: If you are taking blood thinners, such as aspirin, warfarin, or clopidogrel, your doctor will likely advise you to stop these medications several days before surgery to reduce the risk of excessive bleeding.

Diabetes Medications: Patients with diabetes may need to adjust their insulin or oral diabetes medications leading up to surgery. Your healthcare team will provide specific instructions based on your individual needs.

Herbal Supplements: Some herbal supplements, such as garlic, ginkgo biloba, and ginseng, can increase the risk of bleeding or interact with anesthesia. Inform your doctor about any supplements you are taking and follow their advice on whether to discontinue them before surgery.

Pain Medications: Avoid non-steroidal anti-inflammatory drugs (NSAIDs), such as ibuprofen and naproxen, as they can increase the risk of bleeding. Acetaminophen is usually a safer alternative, but always consult your doctor before taking any medication.

Mental preparation is a vital aspect of getting ready for nephrectomy, as it can help reduce anxiety and improve your overall experience and recovery.

Understanding the Procedure: Take the time to learn about the nephrectomy procedure, including the steps involved, potential risks, and expected outcomes. Knowledge can help alleviate fear and provide a sense of control over the situation.

Stress Management Techniques: Practice stress management techniques such as deep breathing exercises, meditation, and mindfulness to help calm your mind and reduce preoperative anxiety. These techniques can also be useful during your recovery.

Support System: Surround yourself with a supportive network of family and friends who can provide emotional support and practical assistance before and after surgery. Don't hesitate to communicate your feelings and concerns with them.

Professional Support: If you are experiencing significant anxiety or emotional distress, consider seeking support from a mental health professional. Counseling or therapy can help you develop coping strategies and address any psychological concerns related to the surgery.

Positive Visualization: Engage in positive visualization techniques by imagining a successful surgery and smooth recovery. Visualizing positive outcomes can help boost your confidence and reduce stress.

Consultation with Healthcare Team

Effective communication with your healthcare team is essential for a successful nephrectomy and smooth recovery.

Preoperative Appointments: Attend all preoperative appointments and follow-up visits as scheduled. These appointments are crucial for discussing the surgical plan, addressing any concerns, and ensuring you are adequately prepared for the procedure.

Ask Questions: Don't hesitate to ask your healthcare team any questions you may have about the surgery, recovery process, or potential complications. Being well-informed can help you feel more confident and at ease.

Follow Instructions: Carefully follow all preoperative instructions provided by your healthcare team, including dietary restrictions, medication adjustments, and lifestyle modifications. Adhering to these guidelines is critical for minimizing surgical risks and optimizing outcomes.

Discuss Anesthesia: Have a detailed discussion with the anesthesiologist about the type of anesthesia that will be used during your nephrectomy. Understanding the anesthesia process and potential side effects can help alleviate concerns and ensure you are well-prepared.

Postoperative Care Plan: Review the postoperative care plan with your healthcare team, including pain management strategies, activity restrictions, and follow-up appointments. Having a clear understanding of what to expect after surgery can help you prepare for a smooth recovery.

CHAPTER FOUR

NEPHRECTOMY SURGERY DAY

What To Expect On Surgery Day

Arriving at the hospital for your nephrectomy can feel overwhelming, but knowing what to expect can ease anxiety. You'll typically check in early in the morning, allowing ample time for pre-operative preparations. Hospital staff will guide you through the registration process, confirming personal details and reviewing your medical history. You'll then be escorted to a pre-operative area where you'll change into a hospital gown.

In the pre-op area, a nurse will take your vital signs—blood pressure, heart rate, and temperature. An intravenous (IV) line will be inserted into your arm to administer fluids and medications. You might also meet with your anesthesiologist, who will discuss your anesthesia plan and address any last-minute questions or concerns. A surgeon may also come by to review the procedure and mark the surgical site.

Once everything is ready, you'll be transported to the operating room on a gurney. This can be a daunting moment, but the surgical team will be there to support you, ensuring you're as comfortable and calm as possible.

Anesthesia Options

Understanding your anesthesia options is crucial for your comfort and safety during nephrectomy. General anesthesia is the most common choice, rendering you completely unconscious and pain-free throughout the surgery. It involves the administration of anesthetic drugs through your IV line and may also include inhalation agents.

In some cases, particularly with less invasive procedures like laparoscopic nephrectomy, regional anesthesia combined with sedation might be an option. This approach involves numbing the specific area of surgery while you're sedated but still somewhat aware. However, this is less common and typically decided based on your overall health, the complexity of the surgery, and your preferences.

The anesthesiologist will discuss the benefits and risks of each option, ensuring you fully understand the chosen method.

They will remain with you throughout the surgery, monitoring your vital signs and adjusting anesthesia levels as needed.

Operating Room Setup

The operating room setup for nephrectomy is meticulously organized to ensure the procedure is conducted smoothly and safely.

Upon entering the operating room, you'll notice a sterile environment with bright lights and various medical equipment. The room is kept at a cooler temperature to maintain a sterile atmosphere.

You'll be moved onto the operating table, which is adjustable to position you correctly for the surgery.

The surgical team, wearing sterile gowns, gloves, and masks, will surround the table. They'll perform a final check, ensuring all necessary instruments and supplies are readily available.

Monitors will be attached to your body to continuously track your vital signs, such as heart rate, blood pressure, and oxygen levels.

Once you're under anesthesia, the surgical team will sterilize the area around your kidney and drape your body with sterile sheets, leaving only the surgical site exposed.

The setup is designed to minimize the risk of infection and ensure the surgeon has the best possible access to your kidney.

The nephrectomy procedure varies depending on whether it's a partial or total nephrectomy and the surgical approach (open, laparoscopic, or robotic). Here's a general step-by-step outline:

Incision: The surgeon makes an incision in your abdomen or side. In laparoscopic or robotic surgery, several small incisions are made instead of one large one.

Accessing the Kidney:

The surgeon carefully moves aside muscles and other tissues to access the kidney. In minimally invasive surgery, specialized instruments and a camera (laparoscope) are used to view and operate on the kidney through small incisions.

Detaching the Kidney: The blood vessels and ureters connected to the kidney are identified and carefully detached. For partial nephrectomy, only the diseased part of the kidney is removed, preserving as much healthy tissue as possible.

Removing the Kidney:

 In a total nephrectomy, the entire kidney is removed. The kidney (or portion) is then extracted through the incision. In laparoscopic surgery, a small bag is used to remove the kidney through one of the small incisions.

Closing The Incision:

Once the kidney is removed, the surgeon will check for bleeding and other issues before closing the incisions with sutures or staples. In minimally invasive surgery, the small incisions are often closed with sutures or surgical glue.

Completion: The surgical area is cleaned, and a sterile dressing is applied. You'll be moved to the recovery area to begin waking up from anesthesia.

After the nephrectomy, you will be moved to a recovery room where nurses will monitor your vital signs and ensure you're waking up from anesthesia without complications.

Pain management begins immediately, typically with medications administered through your IV. You'll be encouraged to start moving gently as soon as possible to prevent complications like blood clots.

The medical team will monitor your urine output to ensure your remaining kidney (or kidneys) is functioning properly. You'll be given clear fluids at first, gradually progressing to solid foods as tolerated. Breathing exercises may be encouraged to prevent lung complications.

Expect to stay in the hospital for a few days, depending on your recovery speed and the type of surgery performed. Nurses will assist you with mobility, helping you get out of bed and walk around. They'll also educate you on how to care for your incisions, manage pain at home, and recognize signs of infection or complications.

Your discharge plan will include detailed instructions on medication, activity restrictions, follow-up appointments, and dietary guidelines.

The initial days after surgery are crucial for recovery, and following your healthcare provider's instructions will help ensure a smooth healing process.

CHAPTER FIVE

RECOVERY PROCESS

Immediate Post-Operative Care

After a nephrectomy, immediate post-operative care is critical for ensuring a smooth recovery. Upon waking from anesthesia, patients are closely monitored in a recovery room where medical staff continuously check vital signs, such as blood pressure, heart rate, and oxygen levels.

This vigilance is crucial to identify any early signs of complications like bleeding or infection.

The surgical site will be dressed, and drainage tubes may be in place to prevent fluid accumulation. These tubes are usually removed within a few days once the drainage decreases. Patients might have a catheter to assist with urination, which is typically removed after a day or two. The nursing team provides regular updates and ensures that patients are comfortable and well-informed about each step of their immediate post-operative care.

Pain management is a priority, and patients are often given pain medication through an intravenous (IV) line. As they stabilize, the transition to oral painkillers is made. Nausea and vomiting can occur due to anesthesia, but anti-nausea medications are available to alleviate these symptoms. The first few days involve minimal movement, primarily resting in bed to allow the body to start healing. However, nurses may encourage gentle leg and foot exercises to promote blood circulation and prevent blood clots.

Pain Management Strategies

Effective pain management is vital for a comfortable recovery after nephrectomy. Pain levels can vary, but most patients experience some degree of discomfort due to the incision and internal healing. Initially, pain relief is administered intravenously, allowing for rapid control of pain. Patient-controlled analgesia (PCA) pumps are often used, enabling patients to administer a controlled dose of pain medication as needed.

As the recovery progresses, the shift from IV to oral pain medication occurs. Nonsteroidal anti-inflammatory drugs (NSAIDs) and acetaminophen are common choices, often combined with opioids for more severe pain. It's essential to follow the prescribed medication regimen and communicate with healthcare providers about any side effects or inadequate pain relief.

Non-pharmacological strategies also play a role in pain management. Techniques such as deep breathing exercises, guided imagery, and relaxation methods can help reduce the perception of pain. Gentle movement and repositioning are encouraged to prevent stiffness and improve comfort. Using supportive pillows to cushion the surgical site while resting can also alleviate discomfort.

Monitoring and follow-up visits are essential components of the nephrectomy recovery process. Post-surgery, patients will have regular check-ups with their healthcare provider to monitor their progress and detect any potential complications early. These visits typically occur within the first few weeks after discharge and continue periodically for several months.

During follow-up visits, the surgical site is examined to ensure proper healing. Healthcare providers check for signs of infection, such as redness, swelling, or discharge.

Blood tests may be conducted to assess kidney function and overall health. Imaging studies, like ultrasounds or CT scans, might be ordered to monitor the remaining kidney's condition and detect any issues that could arise.

Patients are encouraged to keep a log of any symptoms or concerns to discuss during these visits. Common topics include pain levels, changes in urine output, and any new or worsening symptoms.

Open communication with healthcare providers helps tailor the recovery plan and address any complications promptly. Adherence to follow-up schedules is crucial for a successful recovery and long-term health.

Physical Activity And Rehabilitation

Gradual physical activity and rehabilitation are vital to regaining strength and functionality after nephrectomy. In the initial days post-surgery, movement is limited to avoid strain on the surgical site.

However, light activities such as short walks around the hospital room or home are encouraged to promote blood circulation and prevent complications like blood clots.

As recovery progresses, a more structured rehabilitation plan is introduced. This plan includes gentle exercises to improve mobility and strengthen muscles weakened by surgery.

Activities like walking, stretching, and light resistance training are commonly recommended. Patients should follow the guidance of their healthcare team and avoid strenuous activities or heavy lifting until fully cleared by their surgeon.

Physical therapists play a crucial role in the rehabilitation process. They design personalized exercise programs tailored to the patient's recovery stage and overall health.

Regular sessions with a physical therapist can help improve posture, balance, and endurance. Consistency is key, and patients are encouraged to incorporate these exercises into their daily routine to facilitate a faster and smoother recovery.

Diet And Nutrition During Recovery

Proper diet and nutrition are fundamental to supporting the body's healing process after nephrectomy. Initially, patients might experience a reduced appetite or nausea, common side effects of anesthesia and pain medication. Starting with light, easily digestible foods like clear broths, toast, and applesauce can help ease the transition back to regular eating.

As appetite returns, a balanced diet rich in essential nutrients is crucial. Protein is vital for tissue repair and recovery, so incorporating lean meats, fish, eggs, and legumes is beneficial.

Fresh fruits and vegetables provide vitamins and minerals that support overall health and immune function. Staying hydrated is equally important, so drinking plenty of water and avoiding caffeinated or sugary beverages is recommended.

Patients should also be mindful of their kidney function and follow any dietary restrictions provided by their healthcare team.

 For those with reduced kidney function, limiting sodium, potassium, and phosphorus intake may be necessary to avoid overburdening the remaining kidney. Consulting with a dietitian can provide personalized guidance and meal planning to ensure nutritional needs are met while supporting the recovery process.

CHAPTER SIX

POTENTIAL COMPLICATIONS

Undergoing a nephrectomy, whether partial or complete, carries the risk of potential complications. It's essential to be aware of these risks to manage and mitigate them effectively. Potential complications can range from minor issues to more severe conditions.

Bleeding and Infection

One of the primary concerns during and after nephrectomy is the risk of bleeding. Surgeons take meticulous care to control blood loss during the procedure, but post-operative bleeding can still occur.

This can lead to hematomas, which may require further intervention. Another common complication is infection, which can occur at the surgical site or internally.

Signs of infection include fever, increased pain, redness, and discharge at the incision site.

Damage to Surrounding Organs

Given the proximity of the kidneys to other vital organs, there is a risk of accidental damage during surgery.

This could involve the spleen, liver, intestines, or major blood vessels. Surgeons use advanced imaging and careful techniques to minimize this risk, but it's important to understand that such complications, though rare, are possible.

Common Post-Surgical Complications

After a nephrectomy, patients may experience a variety of post-surgical complications. Being informed about these can help in early identification and management.

Pain and Discomfort

Pain is a common issue following surgery, often managed with pain relief medications.

However, persistent or severe pain should not be ignored as it might indicate underlying complications.

Proper pain management plans and gradual movement can aid in reducing discomfort.

Urinary Issues

Post-surgical urinary problems can arise, such as difficulty urinating or changes in urine output and color.

These symptoms might be temporary, but if they persist, they could indicate complications such as urinary tract infections or damage to the urinary tract.

Gastrointestinal Problems

Patients may experience nausea, vomiting, or constipation following surgery, often due to anesthesia, pain medications, or reduced mobility. Maintaining a balanced diet, staying hydrated, and following prescribed medications can help manage these symptoms.

Early Signs Of Complications

Recognizing early signs of complications can significantly improve outcomes. Patients and caregivers should be vigilant and proactive in identifying these symptoms.

Fever and Signs of Infection

A fever might indicate an infection. Patients should monitor their temperature regularly. Signs such as redness, swelling, or pus at the incision site, along with fever, necessitate immediate medical attention.

Abnormal Pain

While some pain is expected, abnormal or severe pain that doesn't improve with medication or new pain in different areas should be reported to a healthcare provider. This could be a sign of internal complications.

Changes in Urine

Alterations in urine color, consistency, or volume can indicate complications. Blood in the urine, for example, is a red flag and should prompt immediate consultation with a healthcare professional.

Managing Complications Effectively

Effective management of complications is crucial for a smooth recovery.

Pain Management

Proper pain management involves not only medications but also techniques such as physical therapy and relaxation exercises.

Patients should follow their healthcare provider's plan strictly and communicate any issues with pain control.

Preventing Infections

To prevent infections, patients should follow strict hygiene practices, keep the surgical site clean and dry, and adhere to any prescribed antibiotic regimens. Any signs of infection should be reported immediately.

Monitoring and Follow-Up

Regular follow-up appointments allow healthcare providers to monitor recovery and address any emerging complications promptly. Patients should keep all scheduled visits and communicate openly about their recovery process.

Long-Term Risks And Considerations

Long-term risks and considerations are important aspects of post-nephrectomy care, impacting a patient's overall health and quality of life.

Reduced Kidney Function

With one kidney removed, the remaining kidney takes on the workload.

Over time, this can lead to reduced kidney function, especially if the remaining kidney becomes damaged. Patients should have regular check-ups to monitor kidney health.

Hypertension

Patients who undergo nephrectomy may be at increased risk for developing high blood pressure. Monitoring blood pressure and adopting a healthy lifestyle, including a balanced diet and regular exercise, can help manage this risk.

Chronic Kidney Disease

The risk of chronic kidney disease (CKD) is higher after nephrectomy. Regular screening for kidney function and early intervention in case of CKD development is essential for maintaining long-term health.

When to Seek Medical Help

Knowing when to seek medical help is critical in preventing minor issues from escalating into serious complications.

Immediate Medical Attention

Patients should seek immediate medical help if they experience severe pain, high fever, significant changes in urine output, or any signs of infection. Prompt intervention can prevent complications from worsening.

Regular Check-Ups

Scheduled follow-up visits are crucial for monitoring recovery and long-term health. Patients should never skip these appointments and should discuss any concerns or unusual symptoms with their healthcare provider.

By understanding potential complications and how to manage them effectively, patients can navigate their recovery with confidence and achieve the best possible outcomes.

CHAPTER SEVEN

LIFE AFTER NEPHRECTOMY

After undergoing a nephrectomy, whether partial or total, adjusting to life with one kidney is a significant aspect of recovery.

Understanding how your body adapts and functions with reduced renal capacity is crucial. Many people find that their remaining kidney compensates remarkably well, allowing them to resume normal activities over time.

Adjusting To Life With One Kidney

Adjusting to life with one kidney involves making some lifestyle changes and being mindful of your health.

Initially, you may experience fatigue or discomfort as your body heals from surgery. It's important to follow your doctor's instructions regarding activity levels and diet to support recovery and maintain kidney function.

Long-Term Health Monitoring

Long-term health monitoring is essential after nephrectomy to ensure your remaining kidney stays healthy.

Regular check-ups with your healthcare provider will involve monitoring kidney function through blood tests and possibly imaging studies. These appointments help detect any potential issues early and allow for timely intervention if needed.

Impact On Daily Activities

The impact of nephrectomy on daily activities varies from person to person. Initially, you may need to limit strenuous activities and gradually increase your activity level as you recover.

Most people find that they can resume their normal daily routines over time, with some adjustments for comfort and safety.

Psychological And Emotional Considerations

Nephrectomy can have psychological and emotional effects, ranging from feelings of loss or anxiety about health to relief from resolving kidney-related issues. It's normal to experience a range of emotions during recovery. Talking to loved ones or a counselor can help process these feelings and adjust to life post-surgery.

Support Resources And Communities

Finding support resources and communities can be invaluable after nephrectomy. Online forums, support groups, and organizations dedicated to kidney health can provide information, encouragement, and practical tips from others who have undergone similar experiences. Connecting with others can help alleviate feelings of isolation and provide a sense of community.

CHAPTER EIGHT

COMMON CONCERNS AND FAQS

Is Nephrectomy Safe?

Nephrectomy, whether partial or complete, is generally considered safe when performed by experienced surgeons in appropriate medical facilities.

The safety of the procedure largely depends on the patient's overall health condition and the reason for the nephrectomy.

Modern surgical techniques and advanced anesthesia contribute significantly to minimizing risks during the procedure.

However, like any surgery, nephrectomy carries some risks, which your healthcare team will discuss with you beforehand to ensure you are well-informed.

How Long Does Recovery Take?

Recovery time after nephrectomy varies based on several factors, including the type of nephrectomy (partial or complete), your overall health, and any complications that may arise during or after surgery. Generally, patients can expect to stay in the hospital for a few days to monitor their recovery and manage any pain or discomfort.

Full recovery can take several weeks to months, during which you may gradually resume normal activities as advised by your healthcare provider. It's essential to follow post-operative care instructions diligently to promote healing and prevent complications.

Will I Need Dialysis After Nephrectomy?

Whether or not you will need dialysis after nephrectomy depends on the remaining kidney's function and your overall health status. In partial nephrectomy, where only a portion of the kidney is removed, the remaining kidney can often compensate adequately without the need for dialysis.

However, in cases of complete nephrectomy or if the remaining kidney has impaired function, dialysis may be necessary.

Your healthcare team will assess your kidney function before and after surgery to determine the need for dialysis and discuss this with you.

Can I Lead A Normal Life After Nephrectomy?

Many patients can lead a normal life after nephrectomy, especially if the procedure was performed to remove a diseased or non-functioning kidney while leaving a healthy kidney intact. After recovery, most individuals can resume regular activities, work, and hobbies.

It's important to maintain a healthy lifestyle, including a balanced diet and regular exercise, to support overall well-being and kidney health. Your healthcare provider will guide any specific lifestyle adjustments based on your circumstances.

What Are The Risks Of Not Having Nephrectomy?

The decision to undergo nephrectomy is often based on the risks of not removing a diseased or damaged kidney.

If left untreated, conditions such as kidney cancer, severe infections, or other kidney diseases can worsen and lead to serious health complications. These may include the spread of cancer, chronic pain, kidney failure, or life-threatening infections.

Your healthcare team will discuss the specific risks associated with your condition and the potential benefits of nephrectomy to help you make an informed decision about your treatment options.

These FAQs aim to provide insight into common concerns surrounding nephrectomy, offering practical information to assist patients and their families in understanding the procedure's implications and outcomes.

CHAPTER NINE

ADVANCES AND FUTURE TRENDS

Advances in nephrectomy techniques have transformed kidney surgery, enhancing both safety and effectiveness for patients worldwide. Minimally invasive approaches, such as laparoscopic and robotic-assisted nephrectomy, represent significant strides in surgical innovation.

These methods involve smaller incisions, reduced blood loss, and faster recovery times compared to traditional open surgery.

The precision afforded by robotic systems, coupled with three-dimensional imaging and enhanced dexterity, allows surgeons to navigate complex anatomical structures with unparalleled accuracy.

Future trends in nephrectomy are poised to further refine these techniques. Ongoing research focuses on improving surgical outcomes through advancements in imaging technology and surgical instrumentation. Innovations like augmented reality guidance systems aim to provide real-time visualization during surgery, optimizing surgical planning and execution.

Additionally, the integration of artificial intelligence holds promise in predicting patient outcomes and personalizing surgical approaches based on individual anatomical variations.

Innovations In Nephrectomy Techniques

Recent innovations in nephrectomy techniques have revolutionized the landscape of kidney surgery, offering patients safer and more effective treatment options.

Traditional open nephrectomy, once the standard of care, has increasingly given way to minimally invasive approaches.

Laparoscopic nephrectomy, for instance, involves several small incisions through which specialized instruments and a camera are inserted. This method minimizes tissue trauma, reduces recovery time, and lowers the risk of postoperative complications.

Robotic-assisted nephrectomy represents a pinnacle of technological advancement in kidney surgery. Utilizing robotic arms controlled by surgeons from a console, this approach offers enhanced precision and maneuverability within the confined space of the body.

High-definition cameras provide magnified, three-dimensional views of the surgical site, enabling surgeons to perform intricate maneuvers with unprecedented accuracy.

Patients undergoing robotic nephrectomy often experience less pain, shorter hospital stays, and quicker return to normal activities compared to traditional surgery.

The field of kidney surgery continues to benefit from robust research and development efforts aimed at improving surgical techniques and patient outcomes. Researchers are exploring novel approaches to nephrectomy, including advancements in tissue preservation, enhanced hemostatic agents, and biocompatible materials for wound closure. These innovations aim to minimize surgical trauma, reduce recovery times, and optimize functional outcomes for patients undergoing kidney surgery.

Cutting-edge imaging technologies play a pivotal role in advancing kidney surgery. Magnetic resonance imaging (MRI) and computed tomography (CT) scans provide detailed preoperative assessments of kidney anatomy, aiding surgeons in planning precise surgical approaches. Real-time intraoperative imaging modalities, such as intraoperative ultrasound and fluorescence-guided surgery, further enhance surgical accuracy and ensure thorough removal of diseased tissue while preserving healthy kidney function.

Potential Future Treatments

The future of nephrectomy holds promise for further advancements in treatment modalities and therapeutic interventions.

Emerging technologies, such as targeted therapies and immunotherapy, show potential in treating kidney cancers and other renal conditions non-invasively. These approaches aim to selectively target cancerous cells while sparing healthy tissue, thereby minimizing the need for extensive surgical intervention.

Nanotechnology represents another frontier in nephrectomy research, offering the possibility of targeted drug delivery and enhanced diagnostic capabilities.

Nanoparticles designed to detect early-stage renal diseases could revolutionize screening protocols, allowing for earlier detection and intervention. Bioengineered kidney tissues and regenerative medicine techniques also hold promise for restoring or replacing damaged kidney function, potentially reducing the necessity for nephrectomy in certain cases.

Improving Outcomes For Patients

Enhancing patient outcomes remains a paramount goal in nephrectomy surgery. Multidisciplinary care teams collaborate to optimize preoperative planning, surgical technique, and postoperative management strategies. Patient-centered approaches focus on personalized care plans tailored to individual needs and preferences, ensuring comprehensive support throughout the surgical journey.

Minimizing surgical complications and promoting faster recovery are central to improving outcomes for nephrectomy patients. Enhanced perioperative care protocols, including optimized pain management strategies and early mobilization protocols, contribute to shorter hospital stays and reduced healthcare costs. Patient education initiatives empower individuals to actively participate in their recovery process, fostering a sense of empowerment and confidence in their postoperative outcomes.

Patient Advocacy And Awareness Efforts

Advocacy and awareness efforts play a pivotal role in supporting patients undergoing nephrectomy and their families.

Patient advocacy organizations collaborate with healthcare providers to educate the public about kidney health, nephrectomy procedures, and available support resources. These initiatives aim to raise awareness about kidney diseases, promote early detection through screening programs, and advocate for improved access to care for all individuals affected by renal conditions.

Support networks and peer-to-peer mentoring programs provide emotional and practical support to patients navigating the challenges of kidney surgery. Patient advocacy groups work tirelessly to advocate for policy changes that enhance kidney disease prevention, research funding, and access to innovative treatment options.

By amplifying patient voices and fostering community engagement, these efforts contribute to a supportive environment where patients feel empowered and informed about their healthcare choices.

9 7 9 8 3 3 3 1 0 7 8 1 7